FITNESS LOG

Name: _____

Telephone: _____

Emergency Contact: _____

Emergency Contact Telephone: _____

LEH▲ANN

Date:

Cardio		
Activity		Time

Weight Training				
Exercise	Weight	Set 1	Set 2	Set 3

Date:

Cardio		
Activity		Time

Weight Training				
Exercise	Weight	Set 1	Set 2	Set 3

Date:

Cardio	
Activity	Time

Weight Training				
Exercise	Weight	Set 1	Set 2	Set 3

Date:

Cardio	
Activity	Time

Weight Training				
Exercise	Weight	Set 1	Set 2	Set 3

Date:

Cardio	
Activity	Time

Weight Training				
Exercise	Weight	Set 1	Set 2	Set 3

Date:

Cardio	
Activity	Time

Weight Training				
Exercice	Weight	Set 1	Set 2	Set 3

Date:

Cardio				
Activity				Time

Weight Training				
Exercise	Weight	Set 1	Set 2	Set 3

Date:

Cardio				
Activity				Time

Weight Training				
Exercise	Weight	Set 1	Set 2	Set 3

Date:

Cardio	
Activity	Time

Weight Training				
Exercise	Weight	Set 1	Set 2	Set 3

Date:

Cardio	
Activity	Time

Weight Training				
Exercise	Weight	Set 1	Set 2	Set 3

Date:

Cardio	
Activity	Time

Weight Training				
Exercise	Weight	Set 1	Set 2	Set 3

Date:

Cardio	
Activity	Time

Weight Training				
Exercise	Weight	Set 1	Set 2	Set 3

Date:

Cardio		
Activity		Time

Weight Training				
Exercise	Weight	Set 1	Set 2	Set 3

Date:

Cardio		
Activity		Time

Weight Training				
Exercise	Weight	Set 1	Set 2	Set 3

Date:				
Cardio				
Activity				Time
Weight Training				
Exercise	Weight	Set 1	Set 2	Set 3

Date:				
Cardio				
Activity				Time
Weight Training				
Exercise	Weight	Set 1	Set 2	Set 3

Date:

Cardio		
Activity		Time

Weight Training				
Exercise	Weight	Set 1	Set 2	Set 3

Date:

Cardio		
Activity		Time

Weight Training				
Exercise	Weight	Set 1	Set 2	Set 3

Date:

Cardio	
Activity	Time

Weight Training				
Exercise	Weight	Set 1	Set 2	Set 3

Date:

Cardio	
Activity	Time

Weight Training				
Exercise	Weight	Set 1	Set 2	Set 3

Date:

Cardio	
Activity	Time

Weight Training				
Exercise	Weight	Set 1	Set 2	Set 3

Date:

Cardio	
Activity	Time

Weight Training				
Exercise	Weight	Set 1	Set 2	Set 3

Date:

Cardio	
Activity	Time

Weight Training				
Exercise	Weight	Set 1	Set 2	Set 3

Date:

Cardio	
Activity	Time

Weight Training				
Exercise	Weight	Set 1	Set 2	Set 3

Date:

Cardio	
Activity	Time

Weight Training				
Exercise	Weight	Set 1	Set 2	Set 3

Date:

Cardio	
Activity	Time

Weight Training				
Exercise	Weight	Set 1	Set 2	Set 3

Date:

Cardio	
Activity	Time

Weight Training				
Exercise	Weight	Set 1	Set 2	Set 3

Date:

Cardio	
Activity	Time

Weight Training				
Exercise	Weight	Set 1	Set 2	Set 3

Date:

Cardio	
Activity	Time

Weight Training				
Exercise	Weight	Set 1	Set 2	Set 3

Date:

Cardio	
Activity	Time

Weight Training				
Exercise	Weight	Set 1	Set 2	Set 3

Date:

Cardio	
Activity	Time

Weight Training				
Exercise	Weight	Set 1	Set 2	Set 3

Date:

Cardio	
Activity	Time

Weight Training				
Exercise	Weight	Set 1	Set 2	Set 3

Date:

Cardio	
Activity	Time

Weight Training				
Exercise	Weight	Set 1	Set 2	Set 3

Date:

Cardio	
Activity	Time

Weight Training				
Exercise	Weight	Set 1	Set 2	Set 3

Date:

Cardio	
Activity	Time

Weight Training				
Exercise	Weight	Set 1	Set 2	Set 3

Date:

Cardio	
Activity	Time

Weight Training				
Exercise	Weight	Set 1	Set 2	Set 3

Date:

Cardio	
Activity	Time

Weight Training				
Exercise	Weight	Set 1	Set 2	Set 3

Date:

Cardio	
Activity	Time

Weight Training				
Exercise	Weight	Set 1	Set 2	Set 3

Date:

Cardio		
Activity		Time

Weight Training				
Exercise	Weight	Set 1	Set 2	Set 3

Date:

Cardio		
Activity		Time

Weight Training				
Exercise	Weight	Set 1	Set 2	Set 3

Date:

Cardio	
Activity	Time

Weight Training				
Exercise	Weight	Set 1	Set 2	Set 3

Date:

Cardio	
Activity	Time

Weight Training				
Exercise	Weight	Set 1	Set 2	Set 3

Date:				
Cardio				
Activity				Time
Weight Training				
Exercise	Weight	Set 1	Set 2	Set 3

Date:				
Cardio				
Activity				Time
Weight Training				
Exercise	Weight	Set 1	Set 2	Set 3

Date:

Cardio	
Activity	Time

Weight Training				
Exercise	Weight	Set 1	Set 2	Set 3

Date:

Cardio	
Activity	Time

Weight Training				
Exercise	Weight	Set 1	Set 2	Set 3

Date:

Cardio	
Activity	Time

Weight Training				
Exercise	Weight	Set 1	Set 2	Set 3

Date:

Cardio	
Activity	Time

Weight Training				
Exercise	Weight	Set 1	Set 2	Set 3

Date:

Cardio		
Activity		Time

Weight Training				
Exercise	Weight	Set 1	Set 2	Set 3

Date:

Cardio		
Activity		Time

Weight Training				
Exercise	Weight	Set 1	Set 2	Set 3

Date:

Cardio	
Activity	Time

Weight Training				
Exercise	Weight	Set 1	Set 2	Set 3

Date:

Cardio	
Activity	Time

Weight Training				
Exercise	Weight	Set 1	Set 2	Set 3

Date:

Cardio	
Activity	Time

Weight Training				
Exercise	Weight	Set 1	Set 2	Set 3

Date:

Cardio	
Activity	Time

Weight Training				
Exercise	Weight	Set 1	Set 2	Set 3

Date:

Cardio	
Activity	Time

Weight Training				
Exercise	Weight	Set 1	Set 2	Set 3

Date:

Cardio	
Activity	Time

Weight Training				
Exercise	Weight	Set 1	Set 2	Set 3

Date:

Cardio		
Activity		Time

Weight Training				
Exercise	Weight	Set 1	Set 2	Set 3

Date:

Cardio		
Activity		Time

Weight Training				
Exercise	Weight	Set 1	Set 2	Set 3

Date:

Cardio	
Activity	Time

Weight Training				
Exercise	Weight	Set 1	Set 2	Set 3

Date:

Cardio	
Activity	Time

Weight Training				
Exercise	Weight	Set 1	Set 2	Set 3

Date:

Cardio		
Activity		Time

Weight Training				
Exercise	Weight	Set 1	Set 2	Set 3

Date:

Cardio		
Activity		Time

Weight Training				
Exercise	Weight	Set 1	Set 2	Set 3

Date:

Cardio		
Activity		Time

Weight Training				
Exercise	Weight	Set 1	Set 2	Set 3

Date:

Cardio		
Activity		Time

Weight Training				
Exercise	Weight	Set 1	Set 2	Set 3

Date:

Cardio	
Activity	Time

Weight Training				
Exercise	Weight	Set 1	Set 2	Set 3

Date:

Cardio	
Activity	Time

Weight Training				
Exercise	Weight	Set 1	Set 2	Set 3

Date:

Cardio		
Activity		Time

Weight Training				
Exercise	Weight	Set 1	Set 2	Set 3

Date:

Cardio		
Activity		Time

Weight Training				
Exercise	Weight	Set 1	Set 2	Set 3

Date:

Cardio	
Activity	Time

Weight Training				
Exercise	Weight	Set 1	Set 2	Set 3

Date:

Cardio	
Activity	Time

Weight Training				
Exercise	Weight	Set 1	Set 2	Set 3

Date:

Cardio	
Activity	Time

Weight Training				
Exercise	Weight	Set 1	Set 2	Set 3

Date:

Cardio	
Activity	Time

Weight Training				
Exercise	Weight	Set 1	Set 2	Set 3

Date:

Cardio	
Activity	Time

Weight Training				
Exercise	Weight	Set 1	Set 2	Set 3

Date:

Cardio	
Activity	Time

Weight Training				
Exercise	Weight	Set 1	Set 2	Set 3

Date:

Cardio	
Activity	Time

Weight Training				
Exercise	Weight	Set 1	Set 2	Set 3

Date:

Cardio	
Activity	Time

Weight Training				
Exercise	Weight	Set 1	Set 2	Set 3

Date:

Cardio	
Activity	Time

Weight Training				
Exercise	Weight	Set 1	Set 2	Set 3

Date:

Cardio	
Activity	Time

Weight Training				
Exercise	Weight	Set 1	Set 2	Set 3

Date:

Cardio	
Activity	Time

Weight Training				
Exercise	Weight	Set 1	Set 2	Set 3

Date:

Cardio	
Activity	Time

Weight Training				
Exercise	Weight	Set 1	Set 2	Set 3

Date:

Cardio		
Activity		Time

Weight Training				
Exercise	Weight	Set 1	Set 2	Set 3

Date:

Cardio		
Activity		Time

Weight Training				
Exercise	Weight	Set 1	Set 2	Set 3

Date:

Cardio	
Activity	Time

Weight Training				
Exercise	Weight	Set 1	Set 2	Set 3

Date:

Cardio	
Activity	Time

Weight Training				
Exercise	Weight	Set 1	Set 2	Set 3

Date:

Cardio	
Activity	Time

Weight Training				
Exercise	Weight	Set 1	Set 2	Set 3

Date:

Cardio	
Activity	Time

Weight Training				
Exercise	Weight	Set 1	Set 2	Set 3

Date:

Cardio	
Activity	Time

Weight Training				
Exercise	Weight	Set 1	Set 2	Set 3

Date:

Cardio	
Activity	Time

Weight Training				
Exercise	Weight	Set 1	Set 2	Set 3

Date:

Cardio	
Activity	Time

Weight Training				
Exercise	Weight	Set 1	Set 2	Set 3

Date:

Cardio	
Activity	Time

Weight Training				
Exercise	Weight	Set 1	Set 2	Set 3

Date:

Cardio	
Activity	Time

Weight Training				
Exercise	Weight	Set 1	Set 2	Set 3

Date:

Cardio	
Activity	Time

Weight Training				
Exercise	Weight	Set 1	Set 2	Set 3

Date:

Cardio	
Activity	Time

Weight Training				
Exercise	Weight	Set 1	Set 2	Set 3

Date:

Cardio	
Activity	Time

Weight Training				
Exercise	Weight	Set 1	Set 2	Set 3

Date:

Cardio	
Activity	Time

Weight Training				
Exercise	Weight	Set 1	Set 2	Set 3

Date:

Cardio	
Activity	Time

Weight Training				
Exercise	Weight	Set 1	Set 2	Set 3

Date:

Cardio		
Activity		Time

Weight Training				
Exercise	Weight	Set 1	Set 2	Set 3

Date:

Cardio		
Activity		Time

Weight Training				
Exercise	Weight	Set 1	Set 2	Set 3

Date:

Cardio	
Activity	Time

Weight Training				
Exercise	Weight	Set 1	Set 2	Set 3

Date:

Cardio	
Activity	Time

Weight Training				
Exercise	Weight	Set 1	Set 2	Set 3

Date:

Cardio	
Activity	Time

Weight Training				
Exercise	Weight	Set 1	Set 2	Set 3

Date:

Cardio	
Activity	Time

Weight Training				
Exercise	Weight	Set 1	Set 2	Set 3

Date:

Cardio	
Activity	Time

Weight Training				
Exercise	Weight	Set 1	Set 2	Set 3

Date:

Cardio	
Activity	Time

Weight Training				
Exercise	Weight	Set 1	Set 2	Set 3

Date:

Cardio	
Activity	Time

Weight Training				
Exercise	Weight	Set 1	Set 2	Set 3

Date:

Cardio	
Activity	Time

Weight Training				
Exercise	Weight	Set 1	Set 2	Set 3

Date:

Cardio	
Activity	Time

Weight Training				
Exercise	Weight	Set 1	Set 2	Set 3

Date:

Cardio	
Activity	Time

Weight Training				
Exercise	Weight	Set 1	Set 2	Set 3

Date:

Cardio	
Activity	Time

Weight Training				
Exercise	Weight	Set 1	Set 2	Set 3

Date:

Cardio	
Activity	Time

Weight Training				
Exercise	Weight	Set 1	Set 2	Set 3

Date:

Cardio	
Activity	Time

Weight Training				
Exercise	Weight	Set 1	Set 2	Set 3

Date:

Cardio	
Activity	Time

Weight Training				
Exercise	Weight	Set 1	Set 2	Set 3

Date:

Cardio	
Activity	Time

Weight Training				
Exercise	Weight	Set 1	Set 2	Set 3

Date:

Cardio	
Activity	Time

Weight Training				
Exercise	Weight	Set 1	Set 2	Set 3

Date:

Cardio	
Activity	Time

Weight Training				
Exercise	Weight	Set 1	Set 2	Set 3

Date:

Cardio	
Activity	Time

Weight Training				
Exercise	Weight	Set 1	Set 2	Set 3

Date:

Cardio	
Activity	Time

Weight Training				
Exercise	Weight	Set 1	Set 2	Set 3

Date:

Cardio	
Activity	Time

Weight Training				
Exercise	Weight	Set 1	Set 2	Set 3

Date:

Cardio	
Activity	Time

Weight Training				
Exercise	Weight	Set 1	Set 2	Set 3

Date:

Cardio	
Activity	Time

Weight Training				
Exercise	Weight	Set 1	Set 2	Set 3

Date:

Cardio	
Activity	Time

Weight Training				
Exercise	Weight	Set 1	Set 2	Set 3

Date:

Cardio	
Activity	Time

Weight Training				
Exercise	Weight	Set 1	Set 2	Set 3

Date:

Cardio	
Activity	Time

Weight Training				
Exercise	Weight	Set 1	Set 2	Set 3

Date:

Cardio	
Activity	Time

Weight Training				
Exercise	Weight	Set 1	Set 2	Set 3

Date:

Cardio	
Activity	Time

Weight Training				
Exercise	Weight	Set 1	Set 2	Set 3

Date:

Cardio	
Activity	Time

Weight Training				
Exercise	Weight	Set 1	Set 2	Set 3

Date:

Cardio	
Activity	Time

Weight Training				
Exercise	Weight	Set 1	Set 2	Set 3

Date:

Cardio	
Activity	Time

Weight Training				
Exercise	Weight	Set 1	Set 2	Set 3

Date:

Cardio	
Activity	Time

Weight Training				
Exercise	Weight	Set 1	Set 2	Set 3

Date:

Cardio	
Activity	Time

Weight Training				
Exercise	Weight	Set 1	Set 2	Set 3

Date:

Cardio	
Activity	Time

Weight Training				
Exercise	Weight	Set 1	Set 2	Set 3

Date:

Cardio	
Activity	Time

Weight Training				
Exercise	Weight	Set 1	Set 2	Set 3

Date:

Cardio	
Activity	Time

Weight Training				
Exercise	Weight	Set 1	Set 2	Set 3

Date:

Cardio	
Activity	Time

Weight Training				
Exercise	Weight	Set 1	Set 2	Set 3

Date:

Cardio				
Activity				Time

Weight Training				
Exercise	Weight	Set 1	Set 2	Set 3

Date:

Cardio				
Activity				Time

Weight Training				
Exercise	Weight	Set 1	Set 2	Set 3

Date:

Cardio	
Activity	Time

Weight Training				
Exercise	Weight	Set 1	Set 2	Set 3

Date:

Cardio	
Activity	Time

Weight Training				
Exercise	Weight	Set 1	Set 2	Set 3

Date:

Cardio	
Activity	Time

Weight Training				
Exercise	Weight	Set 1	Set 2	Set 3

Date:

Cardio	
Activity	Time

Weight Training				
Exercise	Weight	Set 1	Set 2	Set 3

Date:

Cardio		
Activity		Time

Weight Training				
Exercise	Weight	Set 1	Set 2	Set 3

Date:

Cardio		
Activity		Time

Weight Training				
Exercise	Weight	Set 1	Set 2	Set 3

Date:

Cardio	
Activity	Time

Weight Training				
Exercise	Weight	Set 1	Set 2	Set 3

Date:

Cardio	
Activity	Time

Weight Training				
Exercise	Weight	Set 1	Set 2	Set 3

Date:

Cardio	
Activity	**Time**

Weight Training				
Exercise	**Weight**	**Set 1**	**Set 2**	**Set 3**

Date:

Cardio	
Activity	**Time**

Weight Training				
Exercise	**Weight**	**Set 1**	**Set 2**	**Set 3**

Date:

Cardio	
Activity	Time

Weight Training				
Exercise	Weight	Set 1	Set 2	Set 3

Date:

Cardio	
Activity	Time

Weight Training				
Exercise	Weight	Set 1	Set 2	Set 3

Date:

Cardio	
Activity	Time

Weight Training				
Exercise	Weight	Set 1	Set 2	Set 3

Date:

Cardio	
Activity	Time

Weight Training				
Exercise	Weight	Set 1	Set 2	Set 3

Date:

Cardio	
Activity	Time

Weight Training				
Exercise	Weight	Set 1	Set 2	Set 3

Date:

Cardio	
Activity	Time

Weight Training				
Exercise	Weight	Set 1	Set 2	Set 3

Date:

Cardio	
Activity	Time

Weight Training				
Exercise	Weight	Set 1	Set 2	Set 3

Date:

Cardio	
Activity	Time

Weight Training				
Exercise	Weight	Set 1	Set 2	Set 3

Date:

Cardio		
Activity		Time

Weight Training				
Exercise	Weight	Set 1	Set 2	Set 3

Date:

Cardio		
Activity		Time

Weight Training				
Exercise	Weight	Set 1	Set 2	Set 3

Date:

Cardio	
Activity	Time

Weight Training				
Exercise	Weight	Set 1	Set 2	Set 3

Date:

Cardio	
Activity	Time

Weight Training				
Exercise	Weight	Set 1	Set 2	Set 3

Date:

Cardio	
Activity	Time

Weight Training				
Exercise	Weight	Set 1	Set 2	Set 3

Date:

Cardio	
Activity	Time

Weight Training				
Exercise	Weight	Set 1	Set 2	Set 3

Date:

Cardio	
Activity	Time

Weight Training				
Exercise	Weight	Set 1	Set 2	Set 3

Date:

Cardio	
Activity	Time

Weight Training				
Exercise	Weight	Set 1	Set 2	Set 3

Date:

Cardio	
Activity	Time

Weight Training				
Exercise	Weight	Set 1	Set 2	Set 3

Date:

Cardio	
Activity	Time

Weight Training				
Exercise	Weight	Set 1	Set 2	Set 3

Date:

Cardio	
Activity	Time

Weight Training				
Exercise	Weight	Set 1	Set 2	Set 3

Date:

Cardio	
Activity	Time

Weight Training				
Exercise	Weight	Set 1	Set 2	Set 3

Date:

Cardio	
Activity	Time

Weight Training				
Exercise	Weight	Set 1	Set 2	Set 3

Date:

Cardio	
Activity	Time

Weight Training				
Exercise	Weight	Set 1	Set 2	Set 3

Date:

Cardio		
Activity		Time

Weight Training				
Exercise	Weight	Set 1	Set 2	Set 3

Date:

Cardio		
Activity		Time

Weight Training				
Exercise	Weight	Set 1	Set 2	Set 3

Date:

Cardio	
Activity	Time

Weight Training				
Exercise	Weight	Set 1	Set 2	Set 3

Date:

Cardio	
Activity	Time

Weight Training				
Exercise	Weight	Set 1	Set 2	Set 3

Date:

Cardio	
Activity	Time

Weight Training				
Exercise	Weight	Set 1	Set 2	Set 3

Date:

Cardio	
Activity	Time

Weight Training				
Exercise	Weight	Set 1	Set 2	Set 3

Date:

Cardio	
Activity	Time

Weight Training				
Exercise	Weight	Set 1	Set 2	Set 3

Date:

Cardio	
Activity	Time

Weight Training				
Exercise	Weight	Set 1	Set 2	Set 3

Date:

Cardio	
Activity	Time

Weight Training				
Exercise	Weight	Set 1	Set 2	Set 3

Date:

Cardio	
Activity	Time

Weight Training				
Exercise	Weight	Set 1	Set 2	Set 3

Date:

Cardio	
Activity	Time

Weight Training				
Exercise	Weight	Set 1	Set 2	Set 3

Date:

Cardio	
Activity	Time

Weight Training				
Exercise	Weight	Set 1	Set 2	Set 3

Date:

Cardio	
Activity	Time

Weight Training				
Exercise	Weight	Set 1	Set 2	Set 3

Date:

Cardio	
Activity	Time

Weight Training				
Exercise	Weight	Set 1	Set 2	Set 3

Date:

Cardio		
Activity		Time

Weight Training				
Exercise	Weight	Set 1	Set 2	Set 3

Date:

Cardio		
Activity		Time

Weight Training				
Exercise	Weight	Set 1	Set 2	Set 3

Date:

Cardio	
Activity	Time

Weight Training				
Exercise	Weight	Set 1	Set 2	Set 3

Date:

Cardio	
Activity	Time

Weight Training				
Exercise	Weight	Set 1	Set 2	Set 3

Date:

Cardio	
Activity	Time

Weight Training				
Exercise	Weight	Set 1	Set 2	Set 3

Date:

Cardio	
Activity	Time

Weight Training				
Exercise	Weight	Set 1	Set 2	Set 3

Date:

Cardio	
Activity	Time

Weight Training				
Exercise	Weight	Set 1	Set 2	Set 3

Date:

Cardio	
Activity	Time

Weight Training				
Exercise	Weight	Set 1	Set 2	Set 3

Date:

Cardio	
Activity	Time

Weight Training				
Exercise	Weight	Set 1	Set 2	Set 3

Date:

Cardio	
Activity	Time

Weight Training				
Exercise	Weight	Set 1	Set 2	Set 3

Date:

Cardio	
Activity	Time

Weight Training				
Exercise	Weight	Set 1	Set 2	Set 3

Date:

Cardio	
Activity	Time

Weight Training				
Exercise	Weight	Set 1	Set 2	Set 3

Date:

Cardio	
Activity	Time

Weight Training				
Exercise	Weight	Set 1	Set 2	Set 3

Date:

Cardio	
Activity	Time

Weight Training				
Exercise	Weight	Set 1	Set 2	Set 3

Date:

Cardio	
Activity	Time

Weight Training				
Exercise	Weight	Set 1	Set 2	Set 3

Date:

Cardio	
Activity	Time

Weight Training				
Exercise	Weight	Set 1	Set 2	Set 3

Date:

Cardio	
Activity	Time

Weight Training				
Exercise	Weight	Set 1	Set 2	Set 3

Date:

Cardio	
Activity	Time

Weight Training				
Exercise	Weight	Set 1	Set 2	Set 3

Date:

Cardio	
Activity	Time

Weight Training				
Exercise	Weight	Set 1	Set 2	Set 3

Date:

Cardio	
Activity	Time

Weight Training				
Exercise	Weight	Set 1	Set 2	Set 3

Date:

Cardio	
Activity	Time

Weight Training				
Exercise	Weight	Set 1	Set 2	Set 3

Date:

Cardio	
Activity	Time

Weight Training				
Exercise	Weight	Set 1	Set 2	Set 3

Date:

Cardio	
Activity	**Time**

Weight Training				
Exercise	**Weight**	**Set 1**	**Set 2**	**Set 3**

Date:

Cardio	
Activity	**Time**

Weight Training				
Exercise	**Weight**	**Set 1**	**Set 2**	**Set 3**

Date:

Cardio	
Activity	Time

Weight Training				
Exercise	Weight	Set 1	Set 2	Set 3

Date:

Cardio	
Activity	Time

Weight Training				
Exercise	Weight	Set 1	Set 2	Set 3

Date:

Cardio	
Activity	Time

Weight Training				
Exercise	Weight	Set 1	Set 2	Set 3

Date:

Cardio	
Activity	Time

Weight Training				
Exercise	Weight	Set 1	Set 2	Set 3

Date:

Cardio	
Activity	Time

Weight Training				
Exercise	Weight	Set 1	Set 2	Set 3

Date:

Cardio	
Activity	Time

Weight Training				
Exercise	Weight	Set 1	Set 2	Set 3

Date:

Cardio				
Activity				Time

Weight Training				
Exercise	Weight	Set 1	Set 2	Set 3

Date:

Cardio				
Activity				Time

Weight Training				
Exercise	Weight	Set 1	Set 2	Set 3

Date:

Cardio	
Activity	Time

Weight Training				
Exercise	Weight	Set 1	Set 2	Set 3

Date:

Cardio	
Activity	Time

Weight Training				
Exercise	Weight	Set 1	Set 2	Set 3

Date:

Cardio	
Activity	Time

Weight Training				
Exercise	Weight	Set 1	Set 2	Set 3

Date:

Cardio	
Activity	Time

Weight Training				
Exercise	Weight	Set 1	Set 2	Set 3

Date:

Cardio		
Activity		Time

Weight Training				
Exercise	Weight	Set 1	Set 2	Set 3

Date:

Cardio		
Activity		Time

Weight Training				
Exercise	Weight	Set 1	Set 2	Set 3

Date:

Cardio	
Activity	Time

Weight Training				
Exercise	Weight	Set 1	Set 2	Set 3

Date:

Cardio	
Activity	Time

Weight Training				
Exercise	Weight	Set 1	Set 2	Set 3

Date:

Cardio		
Activity		Time

Weight Training				
Exercise	Weight	Set 1	Set 2	Set 3

Date:

Cardio		
Activity		Time

Weight Training				
Exercise	Weight	Set 1	Set 2	Set 3

Date:

Cardio	
Activity	Time

Weight Training				
Exercise	Weight	Set 1	Set 2	Set 3

Date:

Cardio	
Activity	Time

Weight Training				
Exercise	Weight	Set 1	Set 2	Set 3

Date:

Cardio		
Activity		Time

Weight Training				
Exercise	Weight	Set 1	Set 2	Set 3

Date:

Cardio		
Activity		Time

Weight Training				
Exercise	Weight	Set 1	Set 2	Set 3

Date:

Cardio	
Activity	Time

Weight Training				
Exercise	Weight	Set 1	Set 2	Set 3

Date:

Cardio	
Activity	Time

Weight Training				
Exercise	Weight	Set 1	Set 2	Set 3

Date:

Cardio	
Activity	Time

Weight Training				
Exercise	Weight	Set 1	Set 2	Set 3

Date:

Cardio	
Activity	Time

Weight Training				
Exercise	Weight	Set 1	Set 2	Set 3

Date:

Cardio		
Activity		Time

Weight Training				
Exercise	Weight	Set 1	Set 2	Set 3

Date:

Cardio		
Activity		Time

Weight Training				
Exercise	Weight	Set 1	Set 2	Set 3

Date:

Cardio	
Activity	Time

Weight Training				
Exercise	Weight	Set 1	Set 2	Set 3

Date:

Cardio	
Activity	Time

Weight Training				
Exercise	Weight	Set 1	Set 2	Set 3

Date:

Cardio	
Activity	Time

Weight Training				
Exercise	Weight	Set 1	Set 2	Set 3

Date:

Cardio	
Activity	Time

Weight Training				
Exercise	Weight	Set 1	Set 2	Set 3

Date:

Cardio	
Activity	Time

Weight Training				
Exercise	Weight	Set 1	Set 2	Set 3

Date:

Cardio	
Activity	Time

Weight Training				
Exercise	Weight	Set 1	Set 2	Set 3

Date:

Cardio	
Activity	Time

Weight Training				
Exercise	Weight	Set 1	Set 2	Set 3

Date:

Cardio	
Activity	Time

Weight Training				
Exercise	Weight	Set 1	Set 2	Set 3

Date:

Cardio	
Activity	Time

Weight Training				
Exercise	Weight	Set 1	Set 2	Set 3

Date:

Cardio	
Activity	Time

Weight Training				
Exercise	Weight	Set 1	Set 2	Set 3

Date:

Cardio	
Activity	Time

Weight Training				
Exercise	Weight	Set 1	Set 2	Set 3

Date:

Cardio	
Activity	Time

Weight Training				
Exercise	Weight	Set 1	Set 2	Set 3

Date:

Cardio	
Activity	Time

Weight Training				
Exercise	Weight	Set 1	Set 2	Set 3

Date:

Cardio	
Activity	Time

Weight Training				
Exercise	Weight	Set 1	Set 2	Set 3

Date:

Cardio	
Activity	Time

Weight Training				
Exercise	Weight	Set 1	Set 2	Set 3

Date:

Cardio	
Activity	Time

Weight Training				
Exercise	Weight	Set 1	Set 2	Set 3

Notes:

Example:

Date: January 1, 2019				
Cardio				
Activity				Time
Run 5 km				29.45
Weight Training				
Exercise	Weight	Set 1	Set 2	Set 3
Front Fly	8lb	8	8	8
Push-ups	BM	15	15	15
Lat Pullover	20lb	12	12	12
Bench Press	60lb	12	12	12
Tricep Dips	BM	12	12	12
Sit-ups	BM	40	40	40
Bicep Curl	15lb	12	12	12
Deadlift	80lb	10	10	10

www.ingramcontent.com/pod-product-compliance
Lightning Source LLC
Chambersburg PA
CBHW060404290526
45791CB00002B/606